LIFE AFTER CANCER: WHAT THEY DON'T TELL YOU

Keir Whittaker

CONTENTS

Life After Cancer: The Things They Don't Tell You

Introduction

Cancer is a battle unlike any other. It's a fight that tests every part of you—physically, emotionally, and mentally. But what happens after you win? Life after cancer doesn't always go back to what it was before, and while you're no longer in the midst of treatment, new challenges emerge. There are aspects of survivorship that no one prepares you for, things you might not have expected.

This e-book is for those navigating that uncertain space after cancer. Whether you're struggling with lingering physical side effects, emotional ups and downs, or even redefining your relationships and career, this book will explore the things that often go unsaid. It's about living in the aftermath of cancer—not just surviving but finding ways to truly thrive.

Emerging from the shadow of cancer can be both a triumph and a challenge. The end of treatment marks the beginning of a new chapter, one that is often filled with a mix of relief, uncertainty, and complex emotions. This chapter delves into the multifaceted nature of life after cancer, exploring the emotional, physical, and psychological aspects of this transition. Understanding these dynamics is crucial for navigating the post-cancer journey and embracing the opportunities that lie ahead.

The Transition from Treatment to Recovery

The transition from active treatment to recovery is a significant shift that can bring about a range of emotions and adjustments. It's essential to acknowledge and address these changes to facilitate a smoother adjustment to life after cancer.

Emotional Repercussions

- **Post-Treatment Relief and Anxiety**: Completing cancer treatment often brings a sense of relief, but it can also be accompanied by anxiety and fear of recurrence. Understanding that these feelings are normal and expected can help in managing them. Discussing your emotions with a healthcare provider or counselor can offer support and coping strategies.

- **Identity Shifts**: Your identity may have shifted as a result of your cancer experience. You might feel different from who you were before diagnosis. It's important to explore and understand these changes in your sense of self and how they affect your daily life.

Adjusting to New Norms

- **Physical Adjustments**: The physical effects of treatment can linger long after the end of therapy. Issues such as fatigue, changes in body image, and residual pain are common. Addressing these physical changes with your healthcare team and developing a plan for managing them can aid in your recovery.

- **Lifestyle Changes**: Adapting to a new lifestyle that accommodates your post-cancer needs is crucial. This may involve modifications to your diet, exercise routine, and daily activities. Establishing a balanced lifestyle that supports your well-being and health is key to your overall recovery.

Navigating the Psychological Impact

The psychological impact of cancer extends beyond treatment and can significantly influence your post-cancer experience. Addressing these psychological aspects is essential for holistic recovery.

Dealing with Trauma and Stress

- **Post-Traumatic Stress**: Cancer can be a traumatic experience, and its effects may linger. Symptoms such as flashbacks, nightmares, and heightened anxiety can occur. Seeking professional support through therapy or counseling can help you process these experiences and manage stress effectively.

- **Coping with Uncertainty**: The uncertainty of the future can be challenging. Developing coping strategies and focusing on aspects of life you can control can help manage feelings of uncertainty. Mindfulness practices, relaxation techniques, and support groups can provide relief.

Survivor's Guilt

- You made it through, but not everyone does. The feeling of guilt that comes with surviving when others haven't is something many cancer survivors struggle with. It can make you question why you were lucky, why someone else had to lose their battle, and why life still feels heavy when you've "won."
- Coping with survivor's guilt isn't about dismissing these feelings but about learning to accept that you are allowed to be grateful for your life while honouring those who didn't make it. It's important to talk about these feelings with loved ones, support groups, or a therapist. Reaching out for help isn't a sign of weakness; it's part of the healing process.

Fear of Recurrence

- Even after the cancer is gone, a shadow can remain. The fear of cancer coming back is ever-present for many survivors. Every ache, pain, or unfamiliar symptom can send you into a spiral of anxiety, wondering if it's a sign that the cancer has returned.
- Living in constant fear can drain the joy out of life. One way to manage this is through mindfulness—learning to focus on the present moment and not letting fear dictate your actions. Therapy, whether individual or group-based, can also provide tools to help you process these anxieties. Knowing that you're not alone in these fears can be a huge comfort.

Building Resilience

- **Fostering Emotional Resilience**: Building emotional resilience involves developing skills to adapt to life's challenges and bounce back from adversity. Techniques such as positive thinking, problem-solving, and stress management can strengthen your resilience.
- **Setting Realistic Goals**: Setting realistic and achievable goals can provide a sense of purpose and direction. These goals might relate to personal growth, career aspirations, or social connections. Achieving these goals

can enhance your confidence and motivation.

Rebuilding Your Life

- Rebuilding your life after cancer involves creating a new sense of normalcy and purpose. This process can be both empowering and challenging, requiring intentional efforts and self-compassion.

Re-establishing Routines

- **Creating New Routines**: Establishing new routines that accommodate your post-cancer needs can help create stability and structure. This might include incorporating self-care practices, engaging in hobbies, and maintaining social connections.

- **Balancing Priorities**: Reassessing your priorities and finding a balance between personal, professional, and social aspects of life is important. Ensuring that your routines align with your values and goals can contribute to a fulfilling and balanced life.

Embracing New Opportunities

- **Exploring New Interests**: Cancer may have shifted your perspective, leading you to explore new interests and passions. Embracing these opportunities can provide a sense of purpose and excitement. Consider pursuing activities or hobbies that you may not have explored before.

- **Pursuing Personal Growth**: Use your post-cancer experience as an opportunity for personal growth. Reflect on the lessons learned, set new goals, and invest in your personal development. This proactive approach can lead to a more fulfilling and enriched life.

Seeking Support and Resources

- Support and resources are vital components of your recovery journey. Identifying and utilizing these resources can significantly impact your post-cancer experience.

Professional Support

- **Medical Follow-Up**: Regular follow-up appointments with your healthcare team are essential for monitoring your health and addressing any concerns. Ensure that you are keeping up with recommended screenings and check-ups.

- **Therapeutic Support**: Engaging with mental health professionals, such as therapists or counselors, can provide valuable support. Therapy can help you navigate emotional challenges, manage stress, and develop coping strategies.

Community and Social Support

- **Support Groups**: Joining support groups for cancer survivors can offer a sense of community and shared understanding. Connecting with others who have experienced similar challenges can provide emotional support and practical advice.

- **Family and Friends**: Lean on your family and friends for support and encouragement. Open communication about your needs and experiences can strengthen these relationships and provide additional sources of support.

Looking Forward

- As you move forward from cancer treatment, it's important to embrace the opportunities and challenges of this new phase. The journey ahead is one of self-discovery, growth, and renewal.

Embracing a New Chapter

- **Adapting to Change**: Embrace the changes that come with life after cancer. Recognize that this is a new chapter in your life, with its own opportunities and challenges. Adapting to these changes with an open mind and a positive attitude can lead to a fulfilling and meaningful experience.

- **Cultivating Optimism**: Maintaining a sense of optimism

and hope is crucial for navigating the post-cancer journey. Focus on the positive aspects of your life and the potential for new beginnings. Cultivating a positive outlook can enhance your overall well-being and resilience.

Creating a Meaningful Future

- **Defining Your Goals**: Reflect on your aspirations and define goals that align with your values and interests. Creating a meaningful future involves setting intentions and working towards objectives that bring you joy and fulfillment.

- **Living Fully**: Embrace life with a renewed sense of purpose and vitality. Engage in activities that enrich your life, build meaningful relationships, and contribute to your well-being. Living fully involves embracing each moment and making the most of the opportunities that come your way.

CHAPTER 2: PHYSICAL CHANGES NO ONE WARNS YOU ABOUT

After the intense battle with cancer, you're eager to put treatment behind you and move on with your life. But for many survivors, the end of treatment isn't the end of the story. The physical effects of cancer and its treatments can linger long after your doctors have declared you cancer-free. These changes can be unexpected and frustrating, and many survivors feel unprepared for the reality of post-cancer life.

Fatigue and Energy Levels: Learning to Pace Yourself

The exhaustion that comes with cancer-related fatigue is unlike anything most people have experienced. It's not just about being tired at the end of the day—it's a deep, pervasive exhaustion that doesn't go away with sleep or rest. Many survivors find themselves feeling wiped out after doing something as simple as going grocery shopping or even getting dressed.

What makes this fatigue particularly challenging is its unpredictability. You might feel fine one day and completely drained the next, with no clear explanation for the fluctuation. This inconsistency can make it difficult to plan your days, return to work, or engage in social activities.

Practical strategies for managing fatigue include:

- **Energy conservation techniques**: Plan your day around your energy levels. Break tasks into smaller steps and rest between them. If a full day at work is overwhelming, explore the possibility of part-time hours or remote work.

- **Exercise, in moderation**: While it seems counterintuitive, light physical activity like walking, yoga, or swimming can actually help combat fatigue over time. The key is to start small and gradually increase your activity level as your body allows.

- **Sleep hygiene**: Establishing a regular sleep routine can be beneficial. Try to go to bed and wake up at the same time every day and create a restful environment by minimizing noise and light.

It's important to accept that recovery is a long process, and pushing yourself too hard can delay it. Recognize your limits and give yourself permission to rest without guilt.

Changes in Body Image: Coming to Terms with a New Self

The physical toll of cancer treatment - whether it's surgery, chemotherapy, or radiation can leave lasting marks on your body. You may have scars from surgeries, such as a mastectomy, or radiation burns that alter the appearance of your skin. Hair loss, weight gain or loss, and changes in your skin's texture are also common. These changes can be hard to accept, especially when you're already dealing with the emotional aftermath of your illness.

Body image issues aren't just about appearance. They're also about identity. Your body may feel unfamiliar, and this can cause a sense of disconnection. You might avoid mirrors or social situations, feel self-conscious about your scars, or worry about how others will perceive you.

Here are some ways to cope with these challenges:

- **Allow yourself to grieve**: It's okay to mourn the body you had before cancer. Acknowledge that your appearance has changed and give yourself time to process those feelings.

- **Find support**: Talk to other survivors who have gone through similar changes. Hearing how others have adjusted can be reassuring. Many people find online support groups particularly helpful.

- **Take control where you can**: Some survivors find empowerment in making proactive changes to their appearance. This could be wearing wigs, trying out different styles of clothing, or even getting tattoos over scars as a symbol of strength.

- **Seek professional help**: If body image issues become overwhelming, consider seeing a counsellor or therapist who specializes in body dysmorphia or post-cancer recovery. Sometimes, just having someone to talk to can make all the difference.

Lymphedema and Other Long-Term Side Effects: An Ongoing Battle

Lymphedema, a painful swelling caused by the buildup of lymph fluid, is a common but often under-discussed side effect for many cancer survivors, especially those who have had lymph nodes removed or damaged during surgery. The swelling can affect the arms, legs, or other areas, making daily tasks difficult and uncomfortable.

What makes lymphedema particularly frustrating is that it can occur months or even years after treatment, often catching survivors off guard. Managing lymphedema involves compression garments, physical therapy, and sometimes manual lymphatic drainage (a specialized massage technique that helps move lymph fluid). For some, it's a lifelong condition that requires daily management.

Other long-term side effects include:

- **Neuropathy**: Chemotherapy can cause nerve damage, leading to tingling, numbness, or pain in the hands and feet. This can make tasks like buttoning clothes or holding objects difficult.

- **Digestive issues**: Many cancer treatments can cause lasting digestive problems, such as chronic diarrhoea, constipation, or difficulty swallowing.

- **Fertility issues**: Certain cancer treatments, particularly for young people, can affect fertility. Whether it's temporary or permanent, grappling with fertility issues adds another layer of complexity to life after cancer.

While these side effects may not be preventable, being aware of them and proactively managing symptoms can improve your quality of life. It's important to keep an open dialogue with your healthcare team and advocate for follow-up care tailored to your specific needs.

Cognitive Changes ("Chemo Brain"): Finding Clarity in the Fog

"Chemo brain" is a term that survivors use to describe the cognitive difficulties that often follow cancer treatment. It includes memory lapses, difficulty concentrating, and mental fog. These issues can be distressing, especially when you're trying to return to normal activities like work or caring for family members.

While the exact cause of chemo brain is still not fully understood, it's clear that it affects many survivors and can last for months or even years. It can make simple tasks like remembering appointments or multitasking seem insurmountable.

How to manage cognitive changes:

- **Cognitive rehabilitation**: Some cancer centres offer cognitive rehabilitation programs that help survivors improve memory and thinking skills through mental exercises and strategies.

- **Organization tools**: Use calendars, to-do lists, and phone reminders to help you stay on track. Breaking larger tasks into smaller steps can also make them more manageable.

- **Be patient with yourself**: Accept that your brain is healing, just like the rest of your body. Progress might be slow, but with time, many survivors find their cognitive functions improve.

It's essential to remember that "chemo brain" is not a sign of weakness or failure. It's a real and common side effect of treatment, and acknowledging it is the first step toward managing it.

Cancer doesn't just change your body; it changes the dynamics of your relationships, sometimes in ways you didn't anticipate. Your friends, family, and loved ones may have rallied around you during your treatment, but once treatment ends, you're left navigating a new landscape of emotions and interactions. For some, relationships grow stronger, but for others, cancer creates distance and strain. Understanding how these changes impact your relationships and how to manage them can make a significant difference in your post-cancer life.

Family Dynamics Post-Cancer: A New Balance

During your cancer journey, family members may have taken on caregiving roles, putting their own lives on hold to support you. While this support is invaluable, it can create a complex dynamic once treatment is over. The shift from being a patient to a survivor may leave both you and your family unsure of what the "new normal" looks like.

For many survivors, there's an unspoken expectation to bounce back quickly, both physically and emotionally. Family members may assume that once treatment ends, life should return to the way it was before. But the reality is more nuanced. You may still be dealing with lingering side effects, emotional stress, or even a sense of loss for the life you once knew.

How to navigate post-cancer family dynamics:

- **Open communication is crucial**: Let your family know what you're experiencing, both physically and emotionally. Explain that recovery is an ongoing process and that you still need their support, even if you appear "better" on the outside.

- **Acknowledge their feelings**: Caregivers often carry

their own emotional burdens, fear, exhaustion, or even resentment that their lives were disrupted by your illness. Encourage them to express their feelings openly and make space for honest conversations.

- **Redefine roles**: After months or years of being cared for, you may want to reclaim your independence, but this shift can be difficult for family members who've become accustomed to taking care of you. Gradually reintroduce balance into your relationship, allowing them to step back while still offering support when needed.

This transition may be challenging at first, but it's a vital part of moving forward. Patience, empathy, and clear communication can help both you and your family find a new rhythm.

Friendship Challenges: The Surprises of Support (or Lack Thereof)

One of the most surprising aspects of post-cancer life is how friendships can change, often in unexpected ways. Some friends may have been steadfast during your treatment, offering support, meals, or simply being there to listen. Others may have distanced themselves, unsure of how to handle the situation or what to say.

After treatment, some survivors find that their friendships no longer feel the same. You've been through a life-altering experience, and it can be difficult for people who haven't faced cancer to fully understand what you've been through. This can create a sense of isolation, even among close friends.

Navigating post-cancer friendships:

- **Accept that not everyone knows how to respond**: People may pull away not because they don't care, but because they don't know how to handle the intensity of cancer or the changes in you. This isn't an excuse, but understanding their perspective can help you process your feelings.

- **Be selective with your time and energy**: Post-cancer life is about prioritizing the relationships that uplift you. It's okay to let go of friendships that no longer feel supportive or meaningful. Surround yourself with people who understand what you need and are willing to give it.

- **Reconnect or form new bonds**: Cancer can also lead to deep connections with other survivors. Support groups, both in person and online, are places where you can find others who truly understand your experience. These friendships can be incredibly healing, as they're based on a shared understanding of life post-cancer.

It's important to be gentle with yourself as you navigate changing friendships. Not all relationships will survive the transformation you've been through, and that's okay.

Romantic Relationships and Intimacy: Rebuilding Connection

For many survivors, cancer creates a profound shift in romantic relationships, especially when it comes to intimacy. Physical changes from treatment, such as scars, weight loss or gain, and loss of sexual function, can deeply affect how you feel about yourself. Additionally, the emotional toll of your cancer journey can create distance between you and your partner, even if they were supportive during your treatment.

It's common for survivors to experience anxiety or discomfort around intimacy post-cancer. You may worry about your partner's reaction to your changed body or feel disconnected from them after months of focusing solely on survival. At the same time, your partner may be unsure how to reintroduce intimacy after such a traumatic experience.

Steps for navigating intimacy post-cancer:

- **Talk openly about your feelings**: This can be difficult, especially if you feel vulnerable about your body or the emotional distance between you and your partner. However, open communication is essential to rebuilding intimacy. Let your partner know what you're comfortable with and what your concerns are.

- **Take it slow**: Reestablishing physical intimacy doesn't have to happen all at once. Focus on non-sexual forms of affection, such as hand-holding, cuddling, or simply spending quality time together. These small steps can help you rebuild emotional and physical closeness.

- **Consider counselling**: Couples therapy can be incredibly helpful for both partners to process the emotional changes that cancer brings. A therapist can offer strategies for reconnecting and provide a safe space to discuss difficult topics.

It's important to remember that intimacy, like every other aspect of life post-cancer, is a journey. Be patient with yourself and your partner as you navigate this new chapter together.

Parenting After Cancer: Finding Balance

If you're a parent, one of the most challenging aspects of life after cancer is returning to your role as caregiver while still dealing with your own recovery. Whether your children are young or grown, they may have struggled with fear and uncertainty during your illness, and now they're eager to return to "normal" life. However, the reality is that your energy levels, emotions, and priorities may have shifted.

Young children may not fully understand why you're still tired or why you can't always keep up with them, even though the cancer is "gone." Older children or teens may have their own emotional responses, ranging from relief to anger or even withdrawal.

Tips for parenting post-cancer:

- **Be honest with your children**: Age-appropriate honesty is key. Let your children know that while you're no longer sick, your body and mind are still healing.

Reassure them that it's okay to ask questions or express their own fears.

- **Involve them in your recovery**: Depending on their age, children can be a part of your healing process. Invite them to join you for walks, light exercise, or other gentle activities that allow you to bond while respecting your energy levels.

- **Set realistic expectations**: It's easy to feel guilty about not being able to parent the way you did before cancer. But it's important to set realistic expectations for yourself and your children. Explain that some days will be better than others, and that it's okay to ask for help when you need it.

Parenting after cancer requires balancing your children's needs with your own healing. It's a learning process, and it's okay to seek support from friends, family, or a therapist if you're feeling overwhelmed.

In the UK, returning to work or navigating a career after cancer comes with its own set of challenges and opportunities. Whether you're eager to return to your previous job or considering a new career path, understanding your rights as an employee, managing the physical and mental aftermath of treatment, and finding support in the workplace are key to moving forward.

Returning to Work: Balancing Health and Ambition

For many survivors, returning to work is a significant milestone on the road to recovery. It represents a return to normal life, a chance to regain control, and a source of financial stability. However, it's important to pace yourself and recognise that you may need more time and flexibility than you initially expect.

Cancer and its treatment can leave you with lingering fatigue, cognitive challenges, or emotional hurdles. A phased return to work is often the best approach, allowing you to ease back into your responsibilities without overwhelming yourself.

Steps to returning to work successfully:

- **Phased return**: Many UK employers offer phased return-to-work plans. This means gradually increasing your hours and duties over time, rather than jumping straight back into a full workload. Speak to your employer or HR department about creating a tailored plan that takes your recovery into account.

- **Reasonable adjustments**: Under the **Equality Act 2010**, cancer is classified as a disability, which means your employer must make "reasonable adjustments" to help you return to work. These could include flexible hours, reduced workload, remote working, or adjusting your physical workspace to make it more comfortable for you.

- **Keep communication open**: Stay in regular contact with your line manager or HR team. Discuss your progress and any challenges you're facing, so they can continue to support you. Clear communication helps prevent misunderstandings and ensures that any necessary adjustments are made.

It's crucial to be patient with yourself. Your professional identity and confidence may have been affected by your illness, but over time, as your energy and focus return, you'll begin to regain your sense of purpose and ability at work.

Understanding Your Rights as an Employee

In the UK, cancer survivors are protected by a variety of employment laws that ensure you are treated fairly and with dignity upon returning to work.

- **Equality Act 2010**: This legislation recognises cancer as a disability, protecting you from discrimination in the workplace. Your employer cannot treat you less favourably because of your diagnosis, whether that's in terms of pay, promotion, or job security.

- **Reasonable adjustments**: As mentioned, the Equality Act requires employers to make reasonable adjustments to accommodate your health needs. Adjustments could include changes to your hours, duties, or even location of work (for example, allowing you to work from home if commuting is too taxing).

- **Sick leave and Statutory Sick Pay (SSP)**: If you need more time off due to your illness or recovery, you may be entitled to Statutory Sick Pay. SSP is paid for up to 28 weeks, and some employers offer additional sick pay beyond that. Make sure you understand your company's sick pay policy and discuss extended leave options with HR if necessary.

- **Fit notes**: In the UK, if you've been off work for more than seven days, your GP or specialist will need to provide a "fit note" (previously called a sick note) to outline your condition and any recommendations for returning to work, including phased returns or specific adjustments.

Knowing your rights can empower you to advocate for the support you need during your transition back to the workplace.

Managing Cognitive and Physical Challenges at Work

Many cancer survivors in the UK face cognitive issues, often referred to as "chemo brain," which can affect memory, concentration, and problem-solving skills. Additionally, physical side effects like fatigue or neuropathy (nerve damage causing numbness or tingling) can make it difficult to manage the demands of a full workday.

Strategies to manage cognitive and physical challenges:

- **Prioritise and plan**: Use calendars, task lists, and reminders to stay organised. Break down tasks into smaller, manageable steps to avoid feeling overwhelmed. You can use apps or even simple notebooks to help keep track of your workload.

- **Take regular breaks**: Under the **Health and Safety at Work Act 1974**, you are entitled to a safe working environment. Ensure you're taking regular breaks to rest, especially if fatigue or cognitive issues are making it hard to focus. Short, frequent breaks can help reset your mind and body.

- **Flexible working**: The UK has laws around flexible working, and as an employee, you have the right to request a flexible working arrangement. This might mean working fewer hours, adjusting your start and finish times, or working from home. Be open with your employer about your needs.

Remember, it's not about pushing through at all costs. By listening to your body and using the support available to you, you can achieve a more sustainable work-life balance during your recovery.

Exploring New Career Paths: A Fresh Start

After cancer, some people find that their old job no longer feels meaningful or manageable. Your priorities may have shifted, or the experience of illness may have given you a new perspective on life and work. This is a common experience, and for many survivors, it leads to a desire for a fresh start, whether in a new career or a different way of working.

If you're considering a career change, here are some steps to take:

- **Explore your passions**: Take time to think about what truly matters to you now. Cancer often leads survivors to reassess their lives, including their career choices. If your old job no longer aligns with your values, consider exploring work that feels more meaningful.

- **Upskilling and retraining**: In the UK, there are many options for retraining or gaining new qualifications, particularly if you're seeking a career change. You could look into courses offered by organisations like the **Open University**, **FutureLearn**, or **local adult education centres**. There are often government-backed initiatives to help people retrain for new careers.

- **Volunteer work**: If you're unsure about diving straight into a new career, consider volunteering in a field you're interested in. Volunteering can give you a taste of a different industry and help you build new skills and connections without the immediate pressure of a full-time job.

Making a career change after cancer can be empowering and fulfilling. It's an opportunity to realign your work life with your personal values and the new perspectives you've gained.

Support Systems for Cancer Survivors in the Workplace

Navigating work life after cancer doesn't have to be a solitary journey. In the UK, there are numerous resources and support networks available to help you manage the transition.

- **Macmillan Cancer Support**: Macmillan provides a wealth of resources for cancer survivors, including advice on returning to work, understanding your rights, and managing the emotional impact of work after cancer. They also offer a work support service that can help you negotiate with employers and navigate challenges at work.

- **Occupational Health Services**: Many UK employers offer access to Occupational Health Services, which can assess your health and recommend adjustments to your role. This service can be an advocate for your needs, helping to ensure that you're working in a way that supports your recovery.

- **Advisory, Conciliation and Arbitration Service (ACAS)**: ACAS provides free and impartial advice on workplace rights, including how to approach conversations about reasonable adjustments or phased returns. They can also mediate disputes if you feel your employer isn't meeting your needs.

Taking advantage of these resources can make the transition back to work smoother and less stressful. You don't have to do it alone, support is available at every stage of your journey.

CHAPTER 5: EMOTIONAL HEALING AND MENTAL HEALTH

Cancer may be physically behind you, but the emotional aftermath can linger long after treatment ends. Many survivors are surprised by the complexity of emotions they feel - fear, anxiety, grief, and even guilt. This chapter explores the emotional and mental health challenges you may face after beating cancer and provides insights into the support systems available in the UK to help you through the recovery process.

Dealing with Fear of Recurrence: The Anxiety of the 'What If'

One of the most common emotional struggles cancer survivors face is the fear of recurrence. After being given the all-clear, it's normal to experience anxiety about cancer returning. Every ache or unusual symptom can send your mind racing, and follow-up appointments might trigger significant stress. It's important to acknowledge that this fear is natural but shouldn't control your life.

Here's how to manage the fear of recurrence:

- **Acknowledge your feelings**: Accepting that fear is a normal part of survivorship can help you manage it. Don't bottle up your anxiety - talk about it with loved ones or a mental health professional.

- **Stick to a follow-up care plan**: Regular check-ups with your GP or specialist can provide reassurance. Your medical team can track your recovery, help catch any problems early, and address concerns you have about symptoms.

- **Focus on what's in your control**: You can't predict or prevent a recurrence entirely, but living a healthy lifestyle can help reduce the risk. A balanced diet, regular exercise, and managing stress can contribute to your overall well-being. UK-based organisations like **Macmillan Cancer Support** offer resources to help you adopt a healthier post-cancer lifestyle.

- **Mindfulness and relaxation**: Mindfulness practices can be particularly helpful in coping with fear and uncertainty. Simple techniques like deep breathing, yoga, or meditation can help ground you in the present moment and reduce anxiety. You could join local or online mindfulness courses available across the UK, such as those provided by **NHS-approved apps** like Headspace or Calm.

Fear of recurrence is a shadow that might never fully disappear, but you can learn to manage it so that it doesn't overshadow your ability to enjoy life after cancer.

Survivor's Guilt: Why Me?

Another emotional challenge that many survivors encounter is survivor's guilt - the feeling of, *"Why did I survive when others didn't?"* If you've lost friends or fellow patients to cancer, this guilt can weigh heavily. Survivor's guilt is more than just sadness; it can lead to feelings of isolation, depression, or anxiety.

Here's how to cope with survivor's guilt:

- **Acknowledge the guilt**: Guilt is a natural reaction to surviving when others haven't, but it's important to recognise that your survival wasn't something you controlled. Rather than denying the guilt, allow yourself to feel it without judgment.

- **Talk to others**: Speaking about your guilt with other survivors or joining a support group can provide relief. You're not alone in these feelings, and connecting with people who've had similar experiences can be comforting. **Cancer Research UK** and **Macmillan**

Cancer Support both offer survivor support groups and helplines.

- **Find ways to honour those who didn't survive**: Whether through fundraising, advocacy, or simply remembering them in your own way, honouring those who didn't make it can help you channel your emotions into positive action. Many UK charities, like **Cancer Research UK** or **Marie Curie**, offer opportunities to volunteer or participate in fundraising events that make a tangible impact.

Survivor's guilt is a difficult emotion, but by addressing it and finding ways to honour the lives of others, you can begin to navigate through it with greater peace.

Managing Depression and Anxiety

Depression and anxiety are common emotional responses after surviving cancer. The upheaval of your physical health, combined with the emotional stress of treatment and recovery, can lead to a lasting mental health impact. Many survivors feel overwhelmed by feelings of sadness, hopelessness, or worry about the future.

Managing depression and anxiety effectively requires a multi-pronged approach:

- **Seek professional help**: Don't hesitate to reach out to a mental health professional. In the UK, you can access support through your **GP**, who can refer you to counselling or cognitive behavioural therapy (CBT). **NHS services** provide free mental health support, and cancer-specific charities like **Macmillan** also offer counselling services for survivors.

- **Medication**: In some cases, medication might be necessary to manage depression or anxiety. Your GP can discuss whether anti-depressants or anti-anxiety medication could benefit your recovery and how to integrate it into your broader mental health strategy.

- **Talking therapies**: The **NHS's Improving Access to Psychological Therapies (IAPT)** programme is a great resource. It offers free, evidence-based treatments like CBT and counselling. These therapies can help you process the emotional trauma of cancer and develop coping strategies for moving forward.

- **Exercise and physical activity**: Physical activity is not only good for your body, but it can also have a powerful impact on your mental health. Regular exercise releases endorphins that help reduce anxiety and improve mood. Look for low-impact activities like walking, swimming, or yoga, which are often available through **Macmillan's Move More programme**, a UK initiative supporting cancer survivors to get active.

If you feel overwhelmed by emotions after cancer, remember that these feelings are common. By seeking help early and building a strong support network, you can work through the emotional challenges and find your way back to feeling like yourself again.

The Importance of Building a Support Network

Cancer may feel like a solitary battle but building a strong support network is essential for emotional recovery. Surrounding yourself with loved ones, other survivors, or even professional support can provide you with the reassurance and comfort you need as you navigate life after treatment.

Here are some ways to build and strengthen your support network:

- **Friends and family**: The people closest to you are often the first to offer support, but it's important to communicate openly about your needs. Let them know when you need space and when you need company. Sometimes, simply having someone to listen without judgment can be incredibly healing.

- **Peer support groups**: Connecting with other cancer survivors who've been through similar experiences can make you feel less isolated. The UK has a number of organisations, such as **Macmillan, Cancer Research UK**, and **Shine Cancer Support**, which offer peer groups, both in person and online, where you can share your feelings with others who truly understand.

- **Charities and support services**: The UK is home to several excellent cancer support charities. **Maggie's Centres**, located throughout the UK, provide free emotional and practical support for anyone affected by cancer. They offer drop-in sessions, workshops, and counselling in a welcoming, non-clinical setting. Similarly, **Macmillan** provides both online and in-person support, helping survivors navigate the practical and emotional aspects of life after cancer.

A support network doesn't have to be large - it just needs to be meaningful to you. Having people in your corner can make the emotional recovery process smoother and help you feel understood.

Navigating the Emotional Rollercoaster

The emotional journey after cancer is rarely linear. Some days you might feel relieved and optimistic, while other days you might feel overwhelmed by sadness or fear. This is normal, and giving yourself permission to feel all these emotions is key to healing.

Here's how to navigate the ups and downs:

- **Practice self-compassion**: Be kind to yourself. After surviving cancer, it's easy to feel like you should be "over it" and back to normal. But healing - emotionally and physically - takes time. Allow yourself to feel what you need to without guilt or pressure.

- **Set small, achievable goals**: Some days, even small tasks can feel like a victory. Celebrate the little wins - whether it's going for a short walk, cooking a healthy meal, or simply getting out of bed. These small goals can help build momentum towards long-term recovery.

- **Seek professional support when needed**: If you find that you're struggling with persistent feelings of sadness, anxiety, or hopelessness, don't hesitate to reach out to mental health professionals. The UK's **NHS** and cancer charities have a wealth of resources designed to help you process these complex emotions.

One of the biggest yet least discussed impacts of surviving cancer is how it changes your relationships - with partners, family, friends, and even yourself. The emotional and physical toll of cancer often shifts the dynamics of your social life, leaving you to navigate a new landscape in both personal and social spheres.

This chapter will explore how to rebuild, repair, and maintain relationships after cancer, while also managing the unique challenges that come with changes in body image, intimacy, and social interactions.

Rebuilding Relationships with Family and Friends

Your cancer experience may have profoundly affected your relationships with family and friends. While some connections may have grown stronger, others may feel strained or even distant. Often, those closest to you experience their own emotional struggles during your illness and may not know how to support you afterward.

Here's how to navigate and rebuild relationships:

- **Communicate openly**: Post-cancer relationships thrive on open communication. Share your feelings about how your experiences have changed you and encourage your loved ones to express their emotions too. Sometimes, family and friends struggle with their own sense of helplessness during your illness, and having open conversations can bring healing on both sides.

- **Set boundaries**: While support is essential, there may be times when you need space to process your emotions or manage your recovery. It's okay to set boundaries with loved ones, letting them know when you need time to yourself and when you need their company.

- **Acknowledge the changes**: Both you and your loved ones may have changed during your cancer journey. Some people may be more protective or overly cautious, while others may struggle to relate to what you've been through. Acknowledging these changes, rather than ignoring them, can help you work through any tension and rebuild your relationships on a new foundation.

It's also worth exploring family or couple's therapy if certain relationships feel particularly strained. **Relate**, a UK-based organisation, offers relationship counselling to help couples and families navigate these challenges.

Navigating Romantic Relationships and Intimacy

Cancer treatment can significantly impact body image, sexuality, and intimacy. Whether you're in a long-term relationship or dating, it's normal to feel uncertain or anxious about physical and emotional intimacy after cancer. These changes can be particularly challenging if your treatment involved surgeries that altered your body, such as mastectomy, chemotherapy-induced hair loss, or weight changes.

Here are ways to approach intimacy and romantic relationships post-cancer:

- **Body image acceptance**: Cancer can leave lasting scars, both physically and emotionally. Learning to accept your body after treatment is a journey, but it's an important part of regaining confidence in intimate relationships. Speak kindly to yourself and recognise that your body's changes are part of your survival story. In the UK, organisations like **Look Good Feel Better** offer workshops and resources to help cancer survivors rebuild self-confidence and feel comfortable in their own skin.

- **Communicate with your partner**: If you're in a relationship, it's crucial to talk openly with your partner about your concerns or changes in intimacy. Your partner may be unsure how to support you, so expressing your feelings - whether they're about body image, fatigue, or sexual discomfort - can help bridge the gap. Reassure them that intimacy may take time and be patient with each other as you navigate this new reality.

- **Consider professional support**: Sexual issues after cancer are common, and support is available. **Macmillan Cancer Support** provides access to sexual health specialists who can help with physical and emotional barriers to intimacy. The **NHS** also offers sexual health services that can provide advice on regaining a healthy intimate life.

- **Take your time**: Whether you're re-engaging with a long-term partner or entering the dating scene post-cancer, remember that intimacy doesn't need to happen on anyone's timeline but your own. There's no rush to dive back into physical relationships - focus on rebuilding your emotional connection and taking small steps as you feel ready.

For single survivors, dating can feel daunting after cancer. You may wonder how or when to disclose your cancer history. There's no one-size-fits-all approach, but the key is to do what feels right for you - some people choose to share their experiences early on, while others wait until they feel more secure in the relationship. Remember, cancer doesn't define you, and the right person will appreciate and respect your journey.

Social Life After Cancer: Re-entering the World

After surviving cancer, socialising can feel both liberating and overwhelming. You may feel disconnected from friends or uneasy in social situations, especially if your priorities or energy levels have shifted. It's common to feel different from the people around you, who may not fully understand what you've been through.

Here's how to re-enter the social world:

- **Take small steps**: If socialising feels overwhelming, start with small gatherings or one-on-one meetups. This allows you to gradually rebuild your social life at a pace that feels comfortable. You might find that your energy levels fluctuate, so don't feel pressured to attend every social event. Pick and choose based on how you feel.

- **Be honest about your limits**: It's okay to let your friends know that you may need to leave early or take breaks. Most people will be understanding, especially if you explain that your energy levels are still recovering. Setting these expectations can help reduce any social anxiety you might feel about attending events.

- **Reconnect through shared experiences**: If you feel disconnected from your old social circles, it might help to reconnect through shared activities or interests. Whether it's joining a book club, fitness class, or local group, engaging in structured activities can make socialising feel less daunting.

- **Find new social connections**: Your experience with cancer may inspire you to seek out new friendships with people who understand what you've been through. Many UK-based cancer charities, such as **Shine Cancer Support** (which focuses on younger adults affected by cancer), offer peer support groups and social events specifically for survivors. These groups can provide a safe space to share your experiences and connect with others who understand your journey.

Friendships: When They Change or Fade

While cancer can strengthen some friendships, others may change or even fade away. Some friends may have found it difficult to know how to support you during treatment and may still struggle with how to relate to you afterward. This can be a painful realisation, but it's also an opportunity to reassess who brings positivity into your life.

Here's how to cope with changes in friendships:

- **Give it time**: Some friends might need more time to process what you've been through. If a previously close friend has been distant, try reaching out and expressing your feelings. They may not realise how much their absence has affected you and could be open to rebuilding the friendship.

- **Let go when necessary**: Unfortunately, not all friendships survive cancer. Some people may simply not be able to cope with the changes, and that's okay. It's important to prioritise relationships that are supportive and affirming, and to let go of friendships that bring negativity or stress. This can be difficult, but ultimately, your well-being comes first.

- **Celebrate your supportive friends**: Cancer can reveal who your true friends are - those who stick by you through the hard times and celebrate your recovery. Make sure to nurture these friendships, express your gratitude, and continue building strong connections with the people who genuinely support you.

Social Anxiety and Feeling 'Different'

After cancer, it's common to feel like you no longer fit in with your old social circles or activities. You may feel like your experiences have set you apart from your peers, especially if they haven't been through something similar. This feeling of being different can lead to social anxiety or a reluctance to engage with friends and family.

<u>Here's how to manage social anxiety</u>:

- **Be open about your experience**: If you're comfortable, sharing your story with friends can help them understand what you've been through and reduce any feelings of isolation. People are often unsure how to approach cancer survivors, so being open about your experience can break down barriers.

- **Join a support group**: If you're feeling particularly isolated, joining a cancer survivor support group can help you connect with people who truly understand what you're going through. Many UK organisations, such as **Maggie's Centres** and **Macmillan**, offer regular support groups where you can share your experiences in a safe, non-judgmental environment.

- **Practice self-compassion**: It's okay if you feel different - that's part of your journey. Remind yourself that your experiences have given you unique strength and perspective, and it's okay to take time to adjust to social situations. Practice self-compassion and remind yourself that you don't need to be "the same" as you were before cancer to enjoy meaningful relationships.

Surviving cancer often brings a significant shift in your financial landscape. Treatment costs, potential loss of income, and adjustments to your lifestyle can create financial strain. Navigating these changes requires understanding your rights, available support, and practical steps to manage your finances effectively.

Understanding Financial Support Available in the UK

The UK offers a range of financial support options for cancer survivors, designed to help ease the financial burden of treatment and recovery. Familiarising yourself with these resources can alleviate some of the stress associated with managing finances after cancer.

Here's an overview of financial support options available:

- **Statutory Sick Pay (SSP)**: If you're employed and off work due to illness, you may be entitled to SSP. This is paid for up to 28 weeks, and your employer is responsible for arranging it. To qualify, you must be earning above the Lower Earnings Limit and have been off work for at least four consecutive days.

- **Employment and Support Allowance (ESA)**: If you're unable to work due to illness or disability, you might be eligible for ESA. This benefit supports those who are unable to work due to their health condition, and the amount you receive depends on your situation. You can apply online through the **GOV.UK** website.

- **Personal Independence Payment (PIP)**: PIP helps with the extra costs of living with a long-term health condition or disability. It's available to people who have difficulty with daily activities or mobility due to their condition. Eligibility is based on how your condition affects your daily life, rather than the condition itself.

- **Disability Living Allowance (DLA)**: For those who were receiving DLA before the introduction of PIP, you may continue to receive this benefit if you meet the eligibility criteria. DLA is for children under 16 and some adults who need help with personal care or mobility.

- **Macmillan Financial Support**: Macmillan Cancer Support offers practical advice and financial support for people affected by cancer. They can help with applications for benefits, grants, and other financial assistance. Their **Money Advice Service** provides one-to-one support to help you understand and manage your finances.

- **Charitable Grants**: Various charities offer grants to people affected by cancer. For example, **The Royal British Legion**, **Turn2us**, and **The Foyle Foundation** provide financial assistance for cancer survivors. These grants can help with household bills, travel expenses, or other essential costs.

It's essential to explore all available support options to ensure you're receiving the financial help you're entitled to.

Managing Treatment Costs and Expenses

Although the NHS provides free treatment, there are often additional costs associated with cancer care that may not be covered, such as travel expenses, prescription charges, and special dietary needs.

Here's how to manage these costs:

- **Travel costs**: If you need to travel for treatment, you may be eligible for the **NHS Low Income Scheme** or **Patient Travel Costs Scheme**, which can help cover travel expenses. Additionally, **Macmillan Cancer Support** offers a travel expense grant to help with the cost of getting to and from treatment.

- **Prescription charges**: While most cancer medications are available free on the NHS, some prescriptions might still incur charges. If you're on a low income, you might qualify for a **Prescription Prepayment Certificate** or exemption based on your income or medical condition.

- **Special dietary needs**: If your treatment has led to specific dietary needs, you may need to adjust your budget to accommodate these changes. Look into local charities or support groups that offer help with food vouchers or meal services for cancer patients.

Tips for managing these additional expenses:

- **Keep records**: Maintain detailed records of all your medical and travel expenses. This documentation can be helpful when applying for financial support or seeking reimbursement.

- **Budget carefully**: Adjust your budget to account for any additional costs you may incur. Tools like budgeting apps or financial planning software can help you keep track of your spending and identify areas where you might save money.

- **Seek advice**: If managing these expenses feels overwhelming, consider speaking with a financial advisor who specialises in supporting cancer patients. They can provide tailored advice and help you navigate the financial aspects of your recovery.

Adjusting to Changes in Income

Cancer treatment often impacts your ability to work, which can lead to a reduction in income. Whether you've had to reduce your working hours or have been off work entirely, adjusting to these changes requires careful planning.

Here's how to manage changes in income:

- **Assess your financial situation**: Review your income, expenses, and any savings you have. Understanding your financial position will help you make informed decisions about managing your budget and seeking additional support.

- **Explore flexible working options**: If returning to work full-time isn't feasible, consider discussing flexible working options with your employer. This might include reduced hours, remote working, or a phased return to work.

- **Consider new sources of income**: If you're unable to return to your previous job, explore alternative sources of income. This could include part-time work, freelance opportunities, or selling items you no longer need. Websites like **Gumtree** and **eBay** can be useful for selling items and generating extra income.

- **Apply for financial support**: Don't hesitate to apply for financial support if your income has been significantly impacted. Benefits like ESA or PIP can provide a crucial financial cushion during your recovery.

Tips for managing reduced income:

- **Prioritise essential expenses**: Focus on covering essential expenses first, such as housing, utilities, and food. Non-essential spending should be adjusted or postponed until your financial situation stabilises.

- **Seek financial advice**: If you're struggling with budgeting or debt, consider speaking with a financial advisor or debt counsellor. Organisations like

StepChange and **Citizens Advice** offer free, confidential advice to help you manage debt and budget effectively.

Planning for the Future

After cancer, it's essential to plan for both short-term and long-term financial stability. This includes addressing any changes in your financial situation, setting new financial goals, and preparing for potential future needs.

Here's how to plan effectively:

- **Set financial goals**: Determine your financial goals and priorities, whether it's paying off debt, saving for future needs, or building an emergency fund. Setting clear goals will help guide your financial decisions and keep you focused on your long-term objectives.

- **Review your insurance**: Check your insurance policies, including life insurance, critical illness cover, and income protection insurance. Ensure they reflect your current needs and provide adequate coverage in case of future health issues.

- **Update your will**: If you haven't already, consider updating your will and estate plans. Ensuring that your wishes are documented and legally binding will provide peace of mind and ensure your affairs are in order.

Tips for long-term financial planning:

- **Consult a financial advisor**: A financial advisor can help you create a comprehensive financial plan, taking into account your current situation, future goals, and any potential risks. Look for advisors who have experience working with cancer survivors or people with long-term health conditions.

- **Stay informed**: Keep yourself informed about changes in financial support and benefits that may affect you. Regularly review your financial situation and adjust your plan as needed to ensure you remain on track.

Returning to work after cancer can be both a relief and a challenge. Whether you're re-entering your previous job or considering a career change, understanding your rights, managing expectations, and adapting to new realities are crucial steps in this process.

Returning to Work: What You Need to Know

Coming back to work after cancer treatment often involves navigating both logistical and emotional hurdles. It's essential to be aware of your rights and to communicate effectively with your employer to ensure a smooth transition.

Here's how to approach your return to work:

- **Communicate with your employer**: Before returning to work, have an open discussion with your employer about your needs and any adjustments required. You're entitled to request reasonable adjustments under the **Equality Act 2010**, which might include flexible hours, modified duties, or ergonomic changes to your workspace.

- **Plan a phased return**: A phased return to work can help ease you back into your role gradually. This might involve starting with reduced hours or responsibilities and increasing them as you regain strength and confidence. Discuss this option with your employer and your GP.

- **Understand your rights**: The UK law protects you against discrimination due to your health condition. If you face any unfair treatment or discrimination related to your cancer experience, you have the right to raise a grievance or seek advice from organisations such as **Citizens Advice** or **ACAS** (Advisory, Conciliation and Arbitration Service).

Managing Work-Related Stress

Returning to work can be stressful, especially if you're still adjusting to life after cancer. Managing work-related stress is crucial for your overall well-being and successful reintegration into the workplace.

Here's how to manage work-related stress:

- **Set realistic expectations**: Recognise that your energy levels and productivity might fluctuate as you recover. Set realistic goals for yourself and communicate any concerns with your manager. It's important to find a balance that allows you to perform effectively without overextending yourself.

- **Seek support**: Don't hesitate to seek support from your employer or colleagues. Many workplaces offer Employee Assistance Programmes (EAPs) that provide confidential support, including counselling and stress management resources.

- **Practice self-care**: Prioritise self-care to manage stress and maintain your well-being. This includes taking breaks, practising relaxation techniques, and maintaining a healthy work-life balance.

Considering Career Changes

Cancer can prompt you to reassess your career goals and aspirations. You might find that your priorities have shifted, or you may want to explore new career paths that align better with your current situation.

Here's how to navigate a career change:

- **Reflect on your goals**: Take time to reflect on your career goals and what you want from your work life moving forward. Consider what aspects of your job you enjoy and what changes might improve your work experience.

- **Explore new opportunities**: If you're considering a career change, explore opportunities that align with your skills and interests. Look into training programmes, voluntary work, or part-time roles that can help you transition into a new field.

- **Seek professional advice**: Career advisors and coaches can help you navigate a career change. They can offer guidance on job searching, resume writing, and interview preparation. In the UK, organisations such as **National Careers Service** offer free career advice and support.

Understanding Statutory and Workplace Rights

Being informed about your statutory and workplace rights is essential for ensuring fair treatment and protection during your return to work and beyond.

Key rights and protections include:

- **Sick leave and pay**: Understand your entitlement to sick leave and pay, including Statutory Sick Pay (SSP) and any additional sick pay your employer might offer. Familiarise yourself with your company's sickness policy and how it integrates with statutory entitlements.

- **Flexible working**: Under the **Flexible Working**

Regulations 2014, employees with at least 26 weeks of continuous service have the right to request flexible working arrangements. This could include changes to your working hours, location, or job role to accommodate your needs.

- **Reasonable adjustments**: Employers are legally required to make reasonable adjustments to support employees with disabilities, including those recovering from cancer. This could involve changes to your work environment, tasks, or schedule to help you perform your job effectively.

Balancing Work and Health

Maintaining a balance between work and health is crucial for long-term well-being. This balance can be challenging, especially as you adjust to new routines and responsibilities.

Here's how to achieve a healthy work-life balance:

- **Set boundaries**: Establish clear boundaries between work and personal life. This might involve setting specific work hours and creating a dedicated workspace if you're working from home. It's important to make time for relaxation and activities that you enjoy.

- **Monitor your health**: Pay attention to your physical and emotional health. If you notice signs of fatigue or stress, take steps to address them, such as adjusting your workload or seeking support from a healthcare professional.

- **Seek ongoing support**: Regularly review your work situation and health with your employer and healthcare team. If you encounter challenges or need further adjustments, communicate these needs proactively.

Accessing Resources and Support

Navigating the work environment after cancer can be complex, but various resources and support systems are available to help you through this transition.

Useful resources and support include:

- **Macmillan Cancer Support**: Offers resources and advice for cancer survivors returning to work, including guidance on workplace rights and reasonable adjustments.

- **Citizens Advice**: Provides free, confidential advice on employment rights, financial support, and other issues related to cancer recovery.

- **ACAS**: Offers advice on resolving workplace disputes, including issues related to health and disability discrimination.

- **National Careers Service**: Provides career advice and support, including help with career changes and job searching.

Life after cancer presents a unique set of challenges and opportunities. Adjusting to your new reality involves embracing change, prioritising self-care, and fostering personal growth. This chapter delves deeply into how you can navigate this transformative period with resilience and optimism.

Embracing Your New Reality

Adjusting to life after cancer often involves a significant shift in how you view yourself and your life. This period is about understanding and accepting your new normal and finding ways to move forward with confidence.

Understanding and Accepting Change

- **Reflect on Your Journey**: Spend time reflecting on your experience. Consider keeping a journal to document your thoughts, feelings, and milestones. Writing about your journey can help you process your emotions and gain insight into how your experience has shaped you.

- **Acknowledge Your Strengths**: Recognise the resilience and strength you have demonstrated throughout your treatment. Acknowledging these strengths can boost your self-esteem and provide motivation as you adapt to your new circumstances.

- **Redefine Your Identity**: Cancer may have changed how you view yourself. Take time to redefine your identity and what matters most to you. This could involve reassessing your values, goals, and aspirations to align with your new reality.

Finding Joy in the Present

- **Practice Mindfulness**: Mindfulness can help you stay grounded in the present moment. Engage in mindfulness practices such as meditation, deep breathing, or mindful walking. These practices can reduce stress and help you appreciate the present.

- **Celebrate Small Victories**: Recognise and celebrate even the small achievements in your recovery. Whether it's completing a task you struggled with or reaching a personal milestone, celebrating these victories can enhance your sense of accomplishment and joy.

- **Embrace New Experiences**: Explore new activities or hobbies that bring you joy. Engaging in new experiences can provide a sense of purpose and help you connect with your new self.

Prioritising Self-Care

Self-care is essential for maintaining your physical, emotional, and mental well-being. Developing a comprehensive self-care routine tailored to your needs can enhance your overall quality of life.

Physical Self-Care

- **Create a Balanced Diet**: Work with a nutritionist to develop a balanced diet that supports your recovery and overall health. Focus on incorporating a variety of fruits, vegetables, whole grains, and lean proteins. Consider any dietary restrictions or sensitivities you may have developed.

- **Establish a Fitness Routine**: Regular exercise can improve your physical health and boost your mood. Start with gentle activities such as walking or swimming and gradually increase the intensity as your strength improves. Consult with a fitness professional or physiotherapist to design a routine that suits your condition.

- **Ensure Adequate Rest**: Prioritise rest and sleep to support your recovery. Develop a consistent sleep routine and create a restful environment. Avoid stimulating activities before bedtime and consider relaxation techniques such as reading or listening to soothing music.

Emotional and Mental Self-Care

- **Engage in Therapy or Counselling**: Consider speaking with a therapist or counsellor who specialises in cancer recovery or trauma. Therapy can provide a safe space to explore your feelings, develop coping strategies, and address any mental health concerns.

- **Practice Stress Management Techniques**: Incorporate stress management techniques into your routine. Techniques such as progressive muscle relaxation, guided imagery, and yoga can help manage stress and enhance relaxation.

- **Build a Support Network**: Surround yourself with supportive friends and family. Share your experiences and seek emotional support from those who understand your journey. Consider joining a cancer support group to connect with others who have faced similar challenges.

Fostering Personal Growth

Life after cancer offers a unique opportunity for personal growth and self-discovery. Embracing this opportunity can lead to a more fulfilling and enriched life.

Setting and Achieving New Goals

- **Identify New Goals**: Reflect on what you want to achieve in your life moving forward. These goals might relate to personal interests, career aspirations, or relationships. Setting clear, realistic goals can provide direction and motivation.

- **Develop an Action Plan**: Create a detailed action plan for achieving your goals. Break down your goals into manageable steps and set deadlines for each step. This approach can help you stay organised and focused as you work towards your aspirations.

- **Monitor Your Progress**: Regularly review your progress towards your goals. Celebrate your achievements and adjust your plan as needed. Reflect on what you've learned from the process and how it has contributed to your personal growth.

Exploring New Interests and Passions

- **Pursue Hobbies**: Reconnect with old hobbies or explore new interests that bring you joy. Engaging in activities you're passionate about can enhance your sense of purpose and fulfilment.

- **Volunteer or Get Involved**: Consider volunteering for causes you care about. Volunteering can provide a sense of accomplishment and help you connect with others who share your values.

- **Continue Learning**: Take advantage of opportunities for learning and personal development. Enrol in courses, attend workshops, or read books on topics that interest you. Lifelong learning can stimulate your mind and enrich your life.

Building Resilience and Finding Meaning

Cancer survivors often seek to find meaning and purpose in their lives after treatment. Building resilience and finding meaning can help you navigate challenges and live a more fulfilling life.

Building Resilience

- **Develop Coping Strategies**: Build resilience by developing effective coping strategies. Techniques such as cognitive-behavioural therapy (CBT) can help you manage negative thoughts and develop a positive mindset. Practice problem-solving skills and focus on solutions rather than dwelling on challenges.

- **Strengthen Your Support System**: Cultivate strong relationships with supportive individuals. Having a reliable support network can provide emotional strength and practical assistance during difficult times.

- **Practice Self-Compassion**: Be kind to yourself and recognise that it's normal to have setbacks. Practice self-compassion by acknowledging your efforts and treating yourself with understanding and patience.

Finding Meaning and Purpose

- **Reflect on Your Values**: Consider what values and principles are important to you. Reflect on how your experience has shaped these values and how they can guide your actions moving forward.

- **Set Purposeful Goals**: Align your goals with your values and passions. Pursuing goals that resonate with your sense of purpose can provide fulfilment and motivation.

- **Share Your Story**: Consider sharing your cancer journey with others. This could involve writing a blog, giving talks, or participating in support groups. Sharing your story can provide a sense of purpose and inspire others who are facing similar challenges.

Creating a Supportive Environment

Your environment plays a significant role in your overall well-being. Creating a supportive environment that fosters positivity, and comfort can enhance your recovery and personal growth.

Optimising Your Living Space

- **Create a Comfortable Home**: Make your living space a sanctuary by incorporating elements that bring you comfort and joy. This might include comfortable furniture, soothing colours, and personal touches that reflect your personality.

- **Organise Your Space**: Keep your living space organised to reduce stress and promote a sense of calm. Consider decluttering and arranging your belongings in a way that supports your daily routines and activities.

Building Positive Relationships

- **Foster Supportive Connections**: Surround yourself with people who uplift and support you. Build and maintain relationships with individuals who understand and respect your journey.

- **Engage in Community Activities**: Participate in community activities or groups that align with your interests. Engaging with others in a supportive environment can provide a sense of belonging and connection.

Practising Mindfulness and Self-Reflection

- **Incorporate Mindfulness Practices**: Regularly engage in mindfulness practices to enhance your mental and emotional well-being. Mindfulness can help you stay present and manage stress effectively.

- **Engage in Self-Reflection**: Set aside time for self-reflection to evaluate your progress, understand your feelings, and adjust your goals. Self-reflection can provide insight into your personal growth and help you stay aligned with your aspirations.

Looking Forward: Embracing the Future

Embracing the future involves approaching life with hope, optimism, and a willingness to adapt to new circumstances. Your experience with cancer has shaped who you are today, and you have the power to create a fulfilling future.

Cultivating Optimism

- **Focus on Positives**: Train yourself to focus on the positives in your life. Practice gratitude by regularly acknowledging the things you're thankful for. This practice can enhance your outlook and provide motivation.

- **Embrace New Opportunities**: Approach new opportunities with an open mind. Be willing to explore new paths and take risks that align with your values and goals.

Setting Long-Term Aspirations

- **Define Your Vision**: Clarify your vision for the future by identifying long-term aspirations that reflect your passions and values. This vision can guide your decisions and provide a sense of direction.

- **Create a Roadmap**: Develop a roadmap for achieving your long-term aspirations. Outline the steps you need to take and set milestones to track your progress. This roadmap can help you stay focused and motivated.

Celebrating Your Journey

- **Acknowledge Your Growth**: Take time to reflect on and celebrate the growth you've experienced throughout your journey. Recognise the strength and resilience you've demonstrated and the lessons you've learned.

- **Share Your Achievements**: Share your achievements and milestones with others. Celebrating your journey with loved ones can provide a sense of accomplishment and reinforce your progress.

CHAPTER 10: NAVIGATING RELATIONSHIPS AND SOCIAL DYNAMICS

Life after cancer often involves renegotiating relationships and social dynamics. Your experience with cancer can affect how you interact with others and how they perceive and relate to you. Understanding and managing these dynamics is crucial for maintaining healthy relationships and building a supportive social network.

Understanding Changes in Relationships

Cancer can alter your relationships with family, friends, and colleagues. These changes may involve shifts in dynamics, communication patterns, and expectations.

Impact on Family Dynamics

- **Role Changes**: Cancer treatment may have altered family roles and responsibilities. Family members may have taken on additional caregiving duties or adjusted their roles to support you. Recognising these changes and communicating openly can help reestablish balance and understanding.

- **Emotional Strain**: The emotional impact of cancer can affect family relationships. Family members may experience their own stress, anxiety, or grief. Addressing these feelings and seeking family counselling if needed can help improve communication and support within the family.

- **Reconnecting**: Reconnect with family members in meaningful ways. Spend quality time together and engage in activities that strengthen bonds. Openly discuss your needs and feelings to foster mutual understanding and support.

Navigating Friendships

- **Adjusting Expectations**: Your experience with cancer may change how you view and interact with friends. It's important to adjust expectations and communicate openly about your needs and boundaries. Friends may not always know how to support you, so providing guidance can help.

- **Building Supportive Friendships**: Surround yourself with friends who offer genuine support and understanding. Engage with friends who respect your journey and provide a positive, empathetic presence. Consider expressing gratitude for their support and sharing your experiences to deepen your connections.

- **Managing Friendships**: If you encounter friends who are unsupportive or whose responses are hurtful, it's okay to set boundaries or seek new connections. Prioritise relationships that contribute positively to your well-being.

Navigating Social Interactions

- **Handling Conversations**: Conversations about your cancer experience can be challenging. Decide how much detail you want to share and practice responses for common questions or comments. It's okay to set boundaries around discussions if you need to protect your emotional well-being.

- **Managing Social Invitations**: You may find social activities more or less manageable depending on your energy levels and health. Communicate openly with friends and family about your availability and comfort levels. It's okay to decline invitations or modify plans to suit your needs.

- **Building New Social Connections**: Explore new social

opportunities that align with your interests and values. Joining support groups, community organisations, or hobby clubs can help you connect with individuals who share similar experiences and interests.

Communicating Your Needs

Effective communication is key to maintaining healthy relationships and ensuring that your needs are met. Being clear and assertive about your needs can help prevent misunderstandings and build stronger connections.

Expressing Your Needs

- **Be Honest and Open**: Communicate your needs and feelings honestly with those around you. Share your experiences, challenges, and preferences to help others understand your perspective and provide appropriate support.

- **Practice Assertiveness**: Use assertive communication techniques to express your needs without feeling guilty or apologetic. Assertiveness involves clearly stating your needs, listening to others, and finding mutually acceptable solutions.

- **Seek Support**: If you find it challenging to communicate your needs, consider seeking support from a therapist or counsellor. They can help you develop effective communication strategies and address any underlying concerns.

Managing Expectations

- **Set Realistic Expectations**: Recognise that not everyone will understand or respond to your needs in the way you hope. Setting realistic expectations about others' responses can help manage potential disappointments and reduce frustration.

- **Adjust Your Expectations**: Be flexible and willing to adjust your expectations based on the circumstances and the individuals involved. Recognise that relationships may evolve and that adjustments may be necessary for maintaining healthy connections.

Maintaining Boundaries

Setting and maintaining boundaries is essential for protecting your well-being and ensuring that your relationships are supportive and respectful.

Establishing Boundaries

- **Identify Your Boundaries**: Determine what boundaries are necessary for your emotional and physical well-being. This might include limits on how much you share about your experience, the types of support you need, or your availability for social activities.

- **Communicate Clearly**: Clearly communicate your boundaries to others in a respectful and assertive manner. Use "I" statements to express your needs and preferences and be open to discussing any concerns or questions.

Enforcing Boundaries

- **Be Consistent**: Consistently enforce your boundaries to maintain your well-being. If someone crosses a boundary, gently remind them of your needs and preferences. It's important to uphold your boundaries to protect your emotional health.

- **Seek Support if Needed**: If you encounter challenges in maintaining boundaries, seek support from a therapist or support group. They can offer guidance and strategies for navigating difficult conversations and maintaining healthy relationships.

Building a Supportive Social Network

A supportive social network can significantly enhance your well-being and provide a sense of community. Building and nurturing these connections is vital for your recovery and personal growth.

Identifying Supportive Individuals

- **Look for Empathetic Individuals**: Seek out individuals who offer empathy, understanding, and encouragement. These people can provide emotional support and practical assistance as you navigate life after cancer.

- **Cultivate Positive Relationships**: Invest time and energy in relationships that contribute positively to your well-being. Engage with people who uplift and support you and focus on building meaningful connections.

Expanding Your Network

- **Explore Community Resources**: Engage with community resources such as cancer support organisations, local groups, and events. These resources can provide opportunities to connect with others who have similar experiences and interests.

- **Participate in Social Activities**: Join social activities, clubs, or classes that align with your interests. Participating in these activities can help you build new friendships and expand your social network.

Maintaining Healthy Relationships

- **Prioritise Communication**: Maintain open and honest communication with those in your social network. Regularly check in with friends and family and share updates about your life and needs.

- **Express Appreciation**: Show appreciation for the support you receive from others. Expressing gratitude can strengthen relationships and encourage continued support.

Navigating Changes in Professional Relationships

Returning to work or navigating career changes can impact your professional relationships. Managing these dynamics effectively is crucial for maintaining a positive work environment.

Managing Workplace Dynamics

- **Communicate Your Needs**: Clearly communicate any needs or adjustments related to your health or work environment. Discuss these needs with your manager or HR representative to ensure that you receive the support you require.

- **Build Positive Relationships**: Foster positive relationships with colleagues by being approachable, respectful, and supportive. Building a collaborative and positive work environment can enhance your professional experience.

Handling Discrimination or Stigma

- **Know Your Rights**: Be aware of your rights regarding discrimination and stigma in the workplace. The Equality Act 2010 protects individuals from discrimination related to health conditions. If you experience discrimination, seek advice from organisations such as ACAS or Citizens Advice.

- **Seek Support**: If you encounter challenges related to discrimination or stigma, seek support from HR, a mentor, or a professional advisor. Addressing these issues proactively can help maintain a positive work environment.

Finding Fulfilment in Social and Professional Life

Ultimately, finding fulfilment in both your social and professional life involves aligning your activities and relationships with your values, goals, and well-being.

Pursuing Meaningful Activities

- **Identify What Matters Most**: Reflect on what activities and relationships bring you the most satisfaction and fulfilment. Focus on engaging in activities that align with your values and contribute to your sense of purpose.

- **Set Personal and Professional Goals**: Set goals that reflect your aspirations and priorities. Whether personal or professional, these goals should align with your values and contribute to your overall sense of fulfilment.

Balancing Social and Professional Life

- **Prioritise Balance**: Strive for a balance between your social and professional life. Ensure that you allocate time for both personal interests and professional responsibilities in a way that supports your well-being.

- **Adjust as Needed**: Be willing to adjust your balance as circumstances change. Regularly assess your needs and priorities and make adjustments to maintain a fulfilling and balanced life.

After cancer treatment, reclaiming your sense of identity can be a profound journey. The experience may have altered how you view yourself and your place in the world. This chapter explores strategies to reconnect with your sense of self, rediscover your passions, and embrace a renewed identity.

Understanding Changes in Identity

The cancer experience can significantly impact how you perceive yourself and your identity. Recognising and navigating these changes is essential for reclaiming your sense of self.

Reflecting on Your Experience

- **Acknowledge the Impact**: Reflect on how cancer has affected your self-perception and identity. Consider how the experience has shaped your beliefs, values, and priorities. Journaling or talking with a therapist can help you process these changes.

- **Recognise Personal Growth**: Identify the personal growth and strengths you have developed through your journey. Acknowledge the resilience, courage, and adaptability you have demonstrated. Understanding these aspects of your character can help you reconnect with your core identity.

Redefining Your Self-Image

- **Explore New Interests**: Cancer may have changed your interests or passions. Take time to explore new hobbies or revisit old ones. Engaging in activities that bring you joy can help you reconnect with aspects of yourself that may have been overshadowed by your illness.

- **Update Your Self-Concept**: Reevaluate your self-concept and how it aligns with your current reality. Consider how you want to see yourself moving forward and how your experiences have shaped this vision. This may involve redefining your goals, values, and personal identity.

Rediscovering Passions and Interests

Rediscovering what brings you joy, and fulfilment can help you reconnect with your sense of identity and purpose.

Engaging in New Activities

- **Explore New Hobbies**: Take up new hobbies or interests that excite you. This could be anything from learning a new skill, joining a club, or participating in creative projects. Exploring new activities can provide a sense of purpose and pleasure.

- **Revisit Old Passions**: Reconnect with hobbies or interests you enjoyed before your diagnosis. Engaging in activities you loved can help you reclaim parts of your identity that may have been set aside during treatment.

Connecting with Your Community

- **Participate in Community Events**: Join community events or groups that align with your interests and values. Participating in these activities can help you build connections and reinforce your sense of belonging.

- **Volunteer**: Consider volunteering for causes you care about. Volunteering can provide a sense of accomplishment, allow you to contribute to something meaningful, and connect you with like-minded individuals.

Building a Positive Self-Image

Cultivating a positive self-image involves embracing who you are and how you have grown through your experience.

Practice Self-Compassion

- **Be Kind to Yourself**: Treat yourself with kindness and understanding. Recognise that adjusting to life after cancer is a process, and it's okay to have setbacks or challenges. Practice self-compassion by acknowledging your efforts and being gentle with yourself.

- **Challenge Negative Self-Talk**: Address and reframe negative self-talk. When you notice self-critical thoughts, challenge them with positive affirmations and evidence of your strengths and accomplishments.

Celebrate Your Achievements

- **Recognise Your Accomplishments**: Celebrate both big and small achievements in your journey. Reflect on how far you have come and acknowledge the milestones you have reached. Celebrating your successes can boost your confidence and reinforce your sense of identity.

- **Share Your Successes**: Share your achievements with friends, family, or support groups. Sharing your successes can provide a sense of pride and connection with others who understand and support your journey.

Setting and achieving new goals is a vital part of moving forward after cancer. This chapter explores strategies for setting meaningful goals, developing actionable plans, and staying motivated as you work towards your aspirations.

Setting Meaningful Goals

Setting goals that align with your values and aspirations can provide direction and motivation as you move forward.

Identify Your Values and Aspirations

- **Reflect on What Matters**: Consider what is most important to you and what you want to achieve in the future. Reflect on your values, passions, and long-term aspirations. This reflection can help you set goals that are meaningful and aligned with your sense of purpose.

- **Set Specific and Realistic Goals**: Define clear, specific, and achievable goals. Break down larger goals into smaller, manageable steps. Setting realistic goals that are attainable can help you stay focused and motivated.

Develop a Goal-Setting Plan

- **Create an Action Plan**: Develop a detailed action plan for achieving your goals. Outline the steps you need to take, set deadlines, and identify any resources or support you may need. Having a structured plan can help you stay organised and track your progress.

- **Prioritise Your Goals**: Prioritise your goals based on their importance and urgency. Focus on one goal at a time or tackle them in a logical sequence. Prioritising your goals can help you manage your time and energy effectively.

Developing an Action Plan

An actionable plan is essential for making progress towards your goals and achieving success.

Break Down Goals into Steps

- **Define Actionable Steps**: Break down your goals into smaller, actionable steps. Each step should be specific and achievable. This approach can make your goals feel less overwhelming and provide a clear path forward.

- **Set Milestones**: Establish milestones to track your progress. Celebrate these milestones as you reach them to maintain motivation and recognise your achievements.

Establish a Support System

- **Seek Support and Accountability**: Share your goals with supportive friends, family, or mentors. Having an accountability partner can provide encouragement, feedback, and motivation. Regular check-ins with your support system can help you stay on track.

- **Access Resources**: Utilise resources and tools that can assist you in achieving your goals. This might include workshops, online courses, or professional advice. Accessing resources can provide additional support and guidance.

Staying Motivated and Overcoming Challenges

Maintaining motivation and overcoming challenges is crucial for achieving your goals and making progress.

Maintain Motivation

- **Visualise Success**: Use visualization techniques to imagine yourself achieving your goals. Visualising success can enhance your motivation and reinforce your commitment to your goals.
- **Stay Positive**: Cultivate a positive mindset and focus on the progress you are making. Remind yourself of your strengths and achievements to maintain a positive outlook.

Address Challenges

- **Identify Potential Obstacles**: Anticipate potential challenges or obstacles that may arise. Develop strategies for addressing these challenges and adapting your plan as needed.
- **Seek Solutions**: When faced with difficulties, seek solutions and adjust your approach. Problem-solving and resilience are key to overcoming challenges and staying on track.

Reflect and Adjust

- **Review Your Progress**: Regularly review your progress towards your goals. Reflect on what is working well and what may need adjustment. Make any necessary changes to your plan to stay aligned with your objectives.

- **Celebrate Your Successes**: Celebrate your achievements and milestones along the way. Recognising and celebrating your successes can boost your confidence and motivation as you continue working towards your goals.

Cancer can shift your perspective on life in profound ways. Embracing a new perspective involves integrating the lessons learned from your journey into your daily life and future outlook. This chapter explores how to adapt to these changes, find meaning, and live with renewed purpose.

Integrating Lessons Learned

The experience of cancer often teaches valuable life lessons. Integrating these lessons into your perspective can help you live a more meaningful and fulfilled life.

Reflect on Your Journey

- **Identify Key Lessons**: Take time to reflect on the lessons you've learned from your cancer journey. This might include insights about resilience, the importance of relationships, or a deeper understanding of your values. Journaling or discussing these insights with a therapist can help you clarify and integrate them.

- **Apply Lessons to Daily Life**: Consider how you can apply these lessons to your daily life. For example, if you've learned the importance of gratitude, incorporate practices of gratitude into your routine. Applying these lessons can enhance your overall well-being and satisfaction.

Finding Meaning and Purpose

- **Explore Your Purpose**: Reflect on what gives your life meaning and purpose. This might involve pursuing passions, engaging in meaningful work, or contributing to causes that matter to you. Exploring your purpose can help you find direction and motivation.

- **Set Meaningful Goals**: Align your goals with your newfound perspective. Setting goals that reflect your values and aspirations can provide a sense of purpose and fulfilment. These goals might be related to personal growth, relationships, or making a positive impact on others.

Living with Renewed Appreciation

Cancer often leads to a heightened appreciation for life. Embracing this renewed appreciation can enhance your overall quality of life and well-being.

Cultivate Gratitude

- **Practice Gratitude**: Incorporate practices of gratitude into your daily routine. This might include keeping a gratitude journal, expressing appreciation to others, or simply taking time each day to reflect on the positive aspects of your life.

- **Celebrate Life's Moments**: Take time to celebrate and enjoy life's moments, both big and small. Embracing a sense of appreciation for everyday experiences can enhance your overall happiness and satisfaction.

Embrace the Present Moment

- **Practice Mindfulness**: Engage in mindfulness practices to stay present and fully experience each moment. Techniques such as meditation, deep breathing, and mindful activities can help you appreciate the present and reduce stress.

- **Let Go of Regrets**: Focus on the present and let go of regrets about the past. Embracing the present moment can help you build a positive outlook and make the most of your current experiences.

Adapting to Change

Adapting to changes in your life after cancer involves accepting and embracing new realities while maintaining a sense of optimism and resilience.

Embrace Change

- **Accept New Realities**: Recognise and accept the changes that have occurred in your life. This might include physical changes, shifts in relationships, or adjustments in your daily routine. Embracing these changes can help you adapt more effectively.

- **Focus on Growth**: View changes as opportunities for growth and personal development. Embracing a growth mindset can help you navigate transitions and challenges with a positive and proactive attitude.

Build Resilience

- **Develop Coping Strategies**: Build resilience by developing effective coping strategies for managing stress and challenges. This might include seeking support, practicing self-care, and maintaining a positive outlook.

- **Seek Support**: Connect with support groups or individuals who understand your experiences and can offer encouragement and guidance. Building a support network can help you navigate changes and maintain your well-being.

Maintaining your well-being and practicing self-care are essential for living a balanced and fulfilling life after cancer. This chapter delves into strategies for nurturing your physical, emotional, and mental health.

Physical Well-being

Taking care of your physical health is crucial for overall well-being and quality of life.

Adopt a Healthy Lifestyle

- **Eat a Balanced Diet**: Focus on a balanced and nutritious diet that supports your overall health. Incorporate a variety of fruits, vegetables, whole grains, lean proteins, and healthy fats into your meals. Consult with a nutritionist if needed to tailor your diet to your specific needs.

- **Stay Active**: Engage in regular physical activity that suits your abilities and preferences. Exercise can improve your physical fitness, boost your mood, and enhance your overall well-being. Aim for activities you enjoy, such as walking, swimming, or yoga.

Monitor Your Health

- **Keep Up with Medical Appointments**: Regularly attend follow-up appointments and screenings as recommended by your healthcare provider. Monitoring your health helps detect any potential issues early and ensures you receive appropriate care.

- **Listen to Your Body**: Pay attention to your body's signals and adjust your activities and routines accordingly. If you experience any new symptoms or health concerns, seek medical advice promptly.

Emotional and Mental Well-being

Caring for your emotional and mental health is vital for maintaining overall well-being and resilience.

Practice Self-Care

- **Engage in Relaxation Techniques**: Incorporate relaxation techniques into your routine to manage stress and promote emotional well-being. Techniques such as deep breathing, meditation, and progressive muscle relaxation can help reduce anxiety and improve relaxation.

- **Pursue Enjoyable Activities**: Engage in activities that bring you joy and satisfaction. Whether it's a hobby, creative project, or social activity, spending time on activities you enjoy can enhance your emotional well-being.

Seek Emotional Support

- **Connect with Others**: Maintain connections with supportive friends, family, and support groups. Sharing your experiences and feelings with others who understand can provide emotional support and strengthen your social network.

- **Consider Professional Support**: If you experience persistent emotional challenges, consider seeking support from a mental health professional. Therapy or counselling can provide a safe space to explore your feelings and develop coping strategies.

Self-Care Strategies

Incorporating self-care practices into your daily life is essential for maintaining your overall well-being.

Develop a Self-Care Routine

- **Create a Personal Routine**: Develop a self-care routine that includes activities and practices that support your physical, emotional, and mental health. Incorporate activities such as exercise, relaxation, and hobbies into your routine.

- **Prioritise Self-Care**: Make self-care a priority in your life. Set aside dedicated time each day or week for self-care activities and ensure you are taking care of your needs.

Manage Stress and Overwhelm

- **Identify Stressors**: Recognise sources of stress in your life and develop strategies for managing them. This might include setting boundaries, seeking support, or practising stress-reduction techniques.

- **Practice Mindfulness**: Engage in mindfulness practices to manage stress and enhance your overall well-being. Mindfulness can help you stay grounded, reduce anxiety, and improve your emotional resilience.

Building Resilience

Building resilience helps you navigate life's challenges and maintain a positive outlook.

Develop Coping Skills

- **Build Problem-Solving Skills**: Strengthen your problem-solving skills to effectively address challenges and obstacles. Developing effective coping strategies can help you manage stress and maintain resilience.

- **Foster a Supportive Network**: Cultivate a network of supportive individuals who can offer encouragement, advice, and companionship. Building strong connections can enhance your resilience and provide a sense of community.

Maintain a Positive Outlook

- **Focus on Positives**: Cultivate a positive outlook by focusing on the positives in your life and celebrating your achievements. Maintaining a positive perspective can improve your overall well-being and resilience.

- **Practice Gratitude**: Incorporate gratitude practices into your daily life. Recognising and appreciating the positive aspects of your life can enhance your emotional well-being and resilience.

Finding purpose and giving back can provide a deep sense of fulfilment and meaning in life after cancer. This chapter explores how to discover your purpose, engage in activities that align with your values, and contribute to the well-being of others.

Discovering Your Purpose

Finding purpose involves reflecting on your passions, values, and aspirations, and aligning your actions with these insights.

Reflect on Your Passions

- **Identify What Matters**: Reflect on what brings you joy and fulfilment. Consider activities, causes, or goals that resonate with you deeply. Identifying your passions can help you find a sense of purpose and direction.

- **Explore New Interests**: Be open to exploring new interests and experiences. Trying new activities or pursuing new hobbies can help you discover what you are passionate about and how you want to make a difference.

Align Your Actions with Your Values

- **Set Purposeful Goals**: Establish goals that align with your values and aspirations. This might include pursuing a new career path, engaging in volunteer work, or working towards personal growth. Aligning your goals with your values can enhance your sense of purpose.

- **Live with Intention**: Make conscious choices that reflect your values and purpose. Living with intention involves making decisions that align with your goals and contribute to a meaningful and fulfilling life.

Engaging in Meaningful Activities

Participating in activities that align with your purpose and values can provide a sense of accomplishment and satisfaction.

Volunteer Your Time

- **Find Volunteer Opportunities**: Explore volunteer opportunities that align with your interests and values. Volunteering can provide a sense of purpose and allow you to contribute to causes you care about.

- **Make a Difference**: Focus on making a positive impact through your volunteer work. Whether it's supporting a local charity, mentoring others, or participating in community projects, your contributions can make a meaningful difference.

Pursue Personal Projects

- **Engage in Personal Projects**: Take on personal projects or initiatives that align with your passions and goals. This might include creative projects, community outreach, or advocacy work. Pursuing personal projects can provide a sense of fulfilment and achievement.

- **Share Your Story**: Consider sharing your cancer journey and experiences with others. Whether through writing, speaking, or participating in awareness campaigns, sharing your story can inspire and support others facing similar challenges.

Giving Back and Contributing

Contributing to the well-being of others can enhance your own sense of purpose and satisfaction.

Support Others

- **Offer Support**: Provide support and encouragement to others who are facing challenges. Sharing your experiences, offering advice, or simply being a listening ear can make a positive impact on someone's life.

- **Mentor Others**: Consider mentoring individuals who are navigating similar experiences. Your insights and support can provide valuable guidance and encouragement to others in their journey.

Advocate for Change

- **Get Involved in Advocacy**: Engage in advocacy efforts related to cancer awareness, research, or policy changes. Advocating for positive change can help improve the lives of others and contribute to a larger impact.

- **Support Research and Education**: Contribute to cancer research and education efforts through donations, fundraising, or volunteer work. Supporting these initiatives can help advance knowledge and improve outcomes for future generations.

Maintaining a Sense of Fulfilment

Finding and maintaining a sense of fulfilment involves staying connected to your purpose and continuing to engage in meaningful activities.

Reflect Regularly

- **Assess Your Fulfilment**: Regularly reflect on your sense of fulfilment and purpose. Consider how your activities and contributions align with your values and goals. Reflecting on your experiences can help you stay connected to your purpose and make adjustments as needed.

- **Celebrate Achievements**: Celebrate your achievements and contributions. Recognising and celebrating your accomplishments can enhance your sense of fulfilment and motivate you to continue pursuing your goals.

Stay Connected

- **Maintain Engagement**: Stay actively engaged in activities and initiatives that align with your purpose. Continuing to participate in meaningful work and contribute to the well-being of others can provide ongoing fulfilment and satisfaction.

- **Seek New Opportunities**: Be open to new opportunities for growth and contribution. Exploring new ways to engage and make a difference can help you maintain a sense of purpose and continue to find fulfilment in your life.

CONCLUSION: EMBRACING A NEW
CHAPTER IN YOUR LIFE

As you close this book, it's important to reflect on the journey you have undertaken and the new chapter you are about to embrace. Life after cancer is not just about recovery; it's about rediscovery, growth, and moving forward with a renewed sense of purpose and vitality. This conclusion aims to encapsulate the essence of your journey and provide a final perspective on how to navigate this transformative period with resilience and hope.

Reflecting on Your Journey

Your cancer journey has been a profound and transformative experience. It has tested your strength, altered your perspective, and reshaped your sense of self. Reflecting on this journey involves acknowledging both the challenges and the growth you have experienced.

Acknowledge Your Strengths

- **Recognise Your Resilience**: Reflect on the resilience you have demonstrated throughout your diagnosis, treatment, and recovery. Acknowledge the strength and courage it took to face and overcome such a significant challenge. This recognition can reinforce your self-esteem and confidence as you move forward.

- **Celebrate Your Achievements**: Celebrate the milestones you have reached, both big and small. Each achievement, whether it's completing treatment, reclaiming your health, or reaching personal goals, is a testament to your perseverance and dedication.

Embrace the Changes

- **Accept Your New Reality**: Embrace the changes that have occurred as a result of your cancer experience. Accepting these changes and integrating them into your life can help you navigate this new phase with grace and adaptability.

- **Integrate Lessons Learned**: Incorporate the valuable lessons you've learned into your daily life. Whether it's a newfound appreciation for life, a deeper sense of purpose, or a commitment to self-care, integrating these lessons can enhance your well-being and enrich your life.

Moving Forward with Purpose

As you move forward, focusing on purpose and meaningful engagement can provide a sense of direction and fulfilment.

Define Your Goals

- **Set Meaningful Objectives**: Define goals that align with your values and aspirations. Setting objectives that resonate with your sense of purpose can provide motivation and a clear path forward. Whether these goals relate to personal growth, relationships, or contributing to a cause, ensure they reflect your true desires.

- **Create a Plan**: Develop a plan to achieve your goals, outlining actionable steps and setting realistic timelines. A structured approach can help you stay focused and make tangible progress towards your aspirations.

Engage in Meaningful Activities

- **Pursue Passions**: Engage in activities and pursuits that bring you joy and fulfilment. Whether it's a new hobby, volunteer work, or personal projects, finding ways to express your passions can enhance your sense of purpose and satisfaction.

- **Contribute to Others**: Consider how you can give back and contribute to the well-being of others. Whether through volunteering, mentoring, or advocacy, making a positive impact on others can provide a profound sense of fulfilment and connection.

Prioritising Well-being and Self-Care

Maintaining your well-being and practicing self-care are essential for a balanced and fulfilling life after cancer.

Focus on Health

- **Adopt a Healthy Lifestyle**: Continue to prioritise physical health through a balanced diet, regular exercise, and medical check-ups. Maintaining a healthy lifestyle supports your overall well-being and enhances your quality of life.

- **Manage Stress and Emotions**: Practice stress management techniques and seek emotional support as needed. Engaging in relaxation practices, maintaining social connections, and seeking professional guidance can help you manage stress and maintain emotional resilience.

Nurture Relationships

- **Strengthen Connections**: Invest time and effort in building and maintaining meaningful relationships. Open communication, mutual support, and appreciation are key to nurturing strong connections with loved ones.

- **Build New Relationships**: Explore opportunities to connect with new people and expand your social network. Engaging in social activities and joining supportive communities can enrich your life and provide additional support and companionship.

Embracing a New Perspective

Your cancer experience has likely shifted your perspective on life, leading to a renewed appreciation for the present moment and a deeper sense of purpose.

Live with Intention

- **Embrace the Present**: Cultivate mindfulness and appreciation for the present moment. Focusing on the here and now can enhance your overall well-being and allow you to fully experience and enjoy life.

- **Pursue Your Purpose**: Align your actions with your sense of purpose and values. Living with intention involves making choices that reflect your goals and contribute to a meaningful and fulfilling life.

Celebrate Your Journey

- **Acknowledge Your Growth**: Celebrate the growth and transformation that have occurred as a result of your cancer journey. Recognise the strength, resilience, and wisdom you have gained, and embrace the opportunities that lie ahead.

- **Share Your Story**: Consider sharing your experiences and insights with others. Your story can inspire and support those who are navigating similar challenges and contribute to a greater sense of connection and community.

Looking Ahead

As you embark on this new chapter, remember that your journey is unique and personal. Embrace the opportunities for growth, connection, and fulfilment that lie ahead. Moving forward with hope, purpose, and a commitment to your well-being can help you navigate this transformative period with resilience and optimism.

Your story is one of courage, strength, and renewal. May you continue to find joy, purpose, and meaning in every step of your journey. Embrace this new chapter with an open heart and a positive outlook, knowing that you have the power to shape your future and live a life of fulfilment and happiness.

ACKNOWLEDGMENTS

I could not have reached this point without the love, support, and unwavering care of the incredible people around me. First, to my family and friends who stood by me during the most challenging moments—through every appointment, diagnosis, and round of chemo, you were there. You held my hand when I felt weak, lifted my spirits when I was low, and never let me feel alone, even on the darkest days. From the day I almost lost my life to the day I was told I was in remission; you were my rock.

A huge and heartfelt thank you to the many surgeons, specialists, doctors, nurses, and orderlies who cared for me with extraordinary skill and compassion. Your dedication and expertise not only treated my illness but helped me find the strength to keep fighting. I am forever grateful for the brilliant care I received; without you, I would not be sitting here today.

To the carers, both past and present, at Willowcroft Care Home in Waltham Abbey, I owe you all a debt that can never be fully repaid. Venita & Tony Batt, Danielle Duro, Kim Palmer, Frank Pace, Joanne Batho, Catherine McMillan - each of you has made a lasting impact on my life with your kindness and care. There are many more of you, and you know who you are. Thank you for making this place not just a home, but a sanctuary where I could heal and rebuild.

Finally, my deepest gratitude goes to my beloved dog, Sonnie. At 10 years old, you have been my constant companion, offering love, loyalty, and comfort through every stage of this journey. Your presence has been a source of strength and joy when I needed it most.

To all of you, I am eternally thankful.